UNDERSTANDING DISORDERS

WHAT ARE DEVELOPMENTAL DISORDERS?

by Liz Sonneborn

BrightPoint Press

San Diego, CA

BrightPoint Press

an imprint of ReferencePoint Press, Inc.
Printed in the United States

For more information, contact:
BrightPoint Press
PO Box 27779
San Diego, CA 92198
www.BrightPointPress.com

Content Consultant: Rui Peixoto, PhD, Assistant Professor of Psychiatry, University of Pittsburgh

LIBRARY OF CONGRESS CATALOGING-IN-PUBLICATION DATA

Names: Sonneborn, Liz, author.
Title: What are developmental disorders? / by Liz Sonneborn.
Description: San Diego, CA : BrightPoint Press, [2023] | Series: Understanding disorders | Includes bibliographical references and index. | Audience: Grades 10-12
Identifiers: LCCN 2022001702 (print) | LCCN 2022001703 (eBook) | ISBN 9781678204440 (hardcover) | ISBN 9781678204457 (eBook)
Subjects: LCSH: Developmental disabilities--Juvenile literature. | Developmental disabilities--Treatment--Juvenile literature.
Classification: LCC RJ506.D47 S66 2023 (print) | LCC RJ506.D47 (eBook) | DDC 618.92/8588--dc23/eng/20220203
LC record available at https://lccn.loc.gov/2022001702
LC eBook record available at https://lccn.loc.gov/2022001703

CONTENTS

AT A GLANCE

- Developmental disorders may impair learning, behavior, and language. They can also affect the physical body.
- Developmental disorders include intellectual disability (ID), autism spectrum disorder (ASD), attention deficit hyperactivity disorder (ADHD), and specific learning disorder (SLD).
- People with ID struggle with learning and solving problems. They may have trouble taking care of themselves.
- People with ASD find it difficult to communicate with others. They may make repetitive motions.
- People with ADHD have a hard time paying attention and staying still. They find it difficult to focus on tasks and follow instructions.
- People with SLD may have difficulties with reading, writing, or doing math.

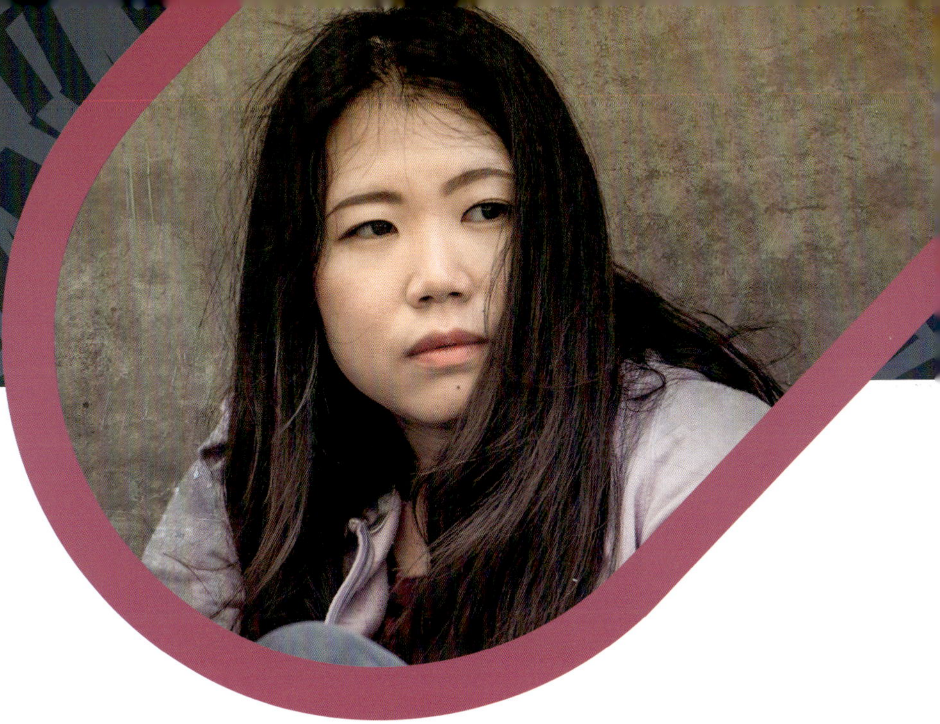

- There are many causes of developmental disorders. They include genetics, toxins, and problems during pregnancy.
- Some symptoms of ADHD can be treated with medication. The symptoms of other disorders can be managed through various therapies and special education.
- Symptoms of developmental disorders can be severe. They may not improve with treatments that are currently available.

BEING DIFFERENT IS A SUPERPOWER

At age eleven, Greta Thunberg felt alone in the world. The Swedish girl had no friends. Other kids said she acted weird. They pushed her down on the playground. Greta became depressed. She cried every day. She stopped talking. She had very little appetite.

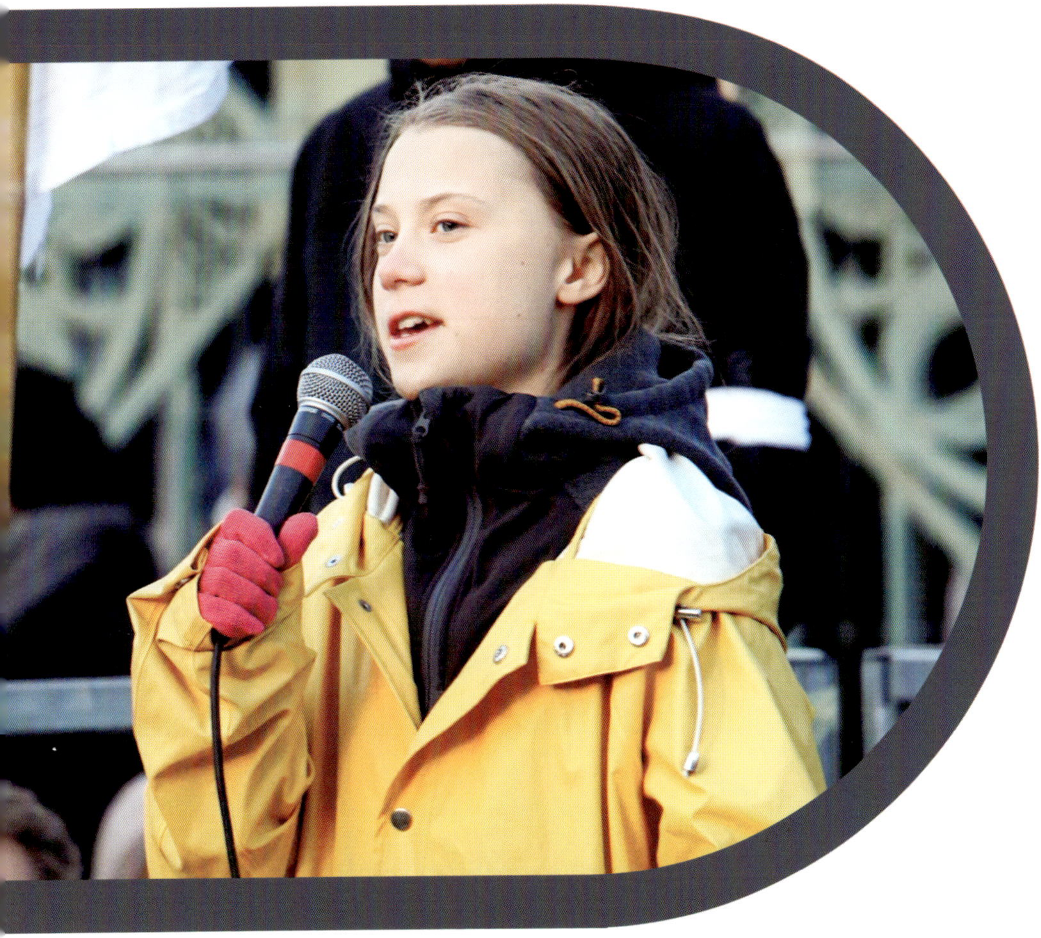

Climate activist Greta Thunberg has spoken about being on the autism spectrum.

Greta was also worried about the environment. In school, she had learned about climate change. The climate was warming due to the burning of fossil fuels, such as oil. Greta was afraid that people were destroying the earth. And it seemed like no one cared but her.

Greta was later **diagnosed** with mild autism spectrum disorder (ASD). ASD explained much of her unhappiness. ASD affects social skills. Greta said whatever she meant directly. That made her seem strange to her bullies. Autism also explained her obsession with climate change. People with ASD can be very focused on their interests.

That focus helped Greta out of her depression. In August 2018, fifteen-year-old Greta started a protest. She skipped school

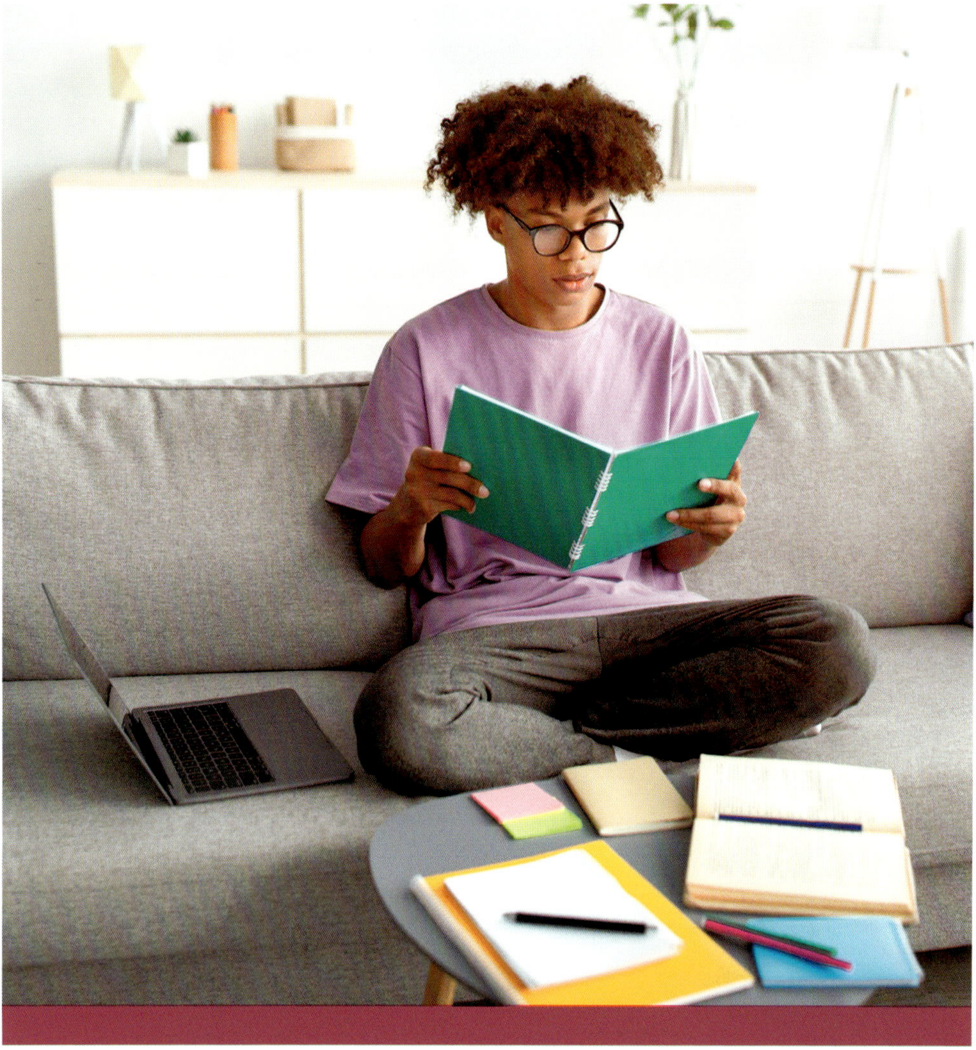

Someone with ASD may be able to focus deeply on subjects that are interesting to him.

and spent the day outside the Swedish Parliament. She held a sign that read "School Strike for Climate." In September

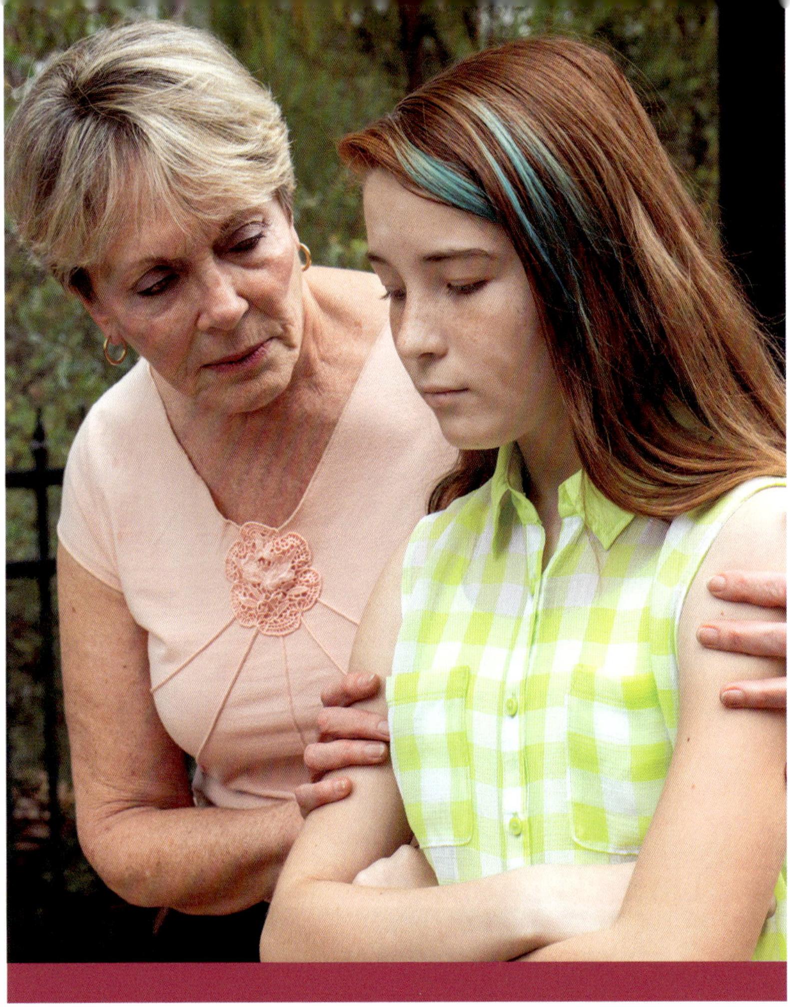

A person with ASD may struggle with eye contact.

2019, 4 million people joined her as part of a strike against climate change. The strike attracted international attention.

Greta has also spoken about her autism diagnosis. In a tweet, she wrote, "I have [autism], and that means I'm sometimes a bit different from the norm." She added, "And, given the right circumstances, being different is a superpower."[1] Autism had caused problems in Greta's life. But it had also helped her start a worldwide movement.

ABOUT DEVELOPMENTAL DISORDERS

Like Greta, millions of people worldwide have developmental disorders, which include ASD. These disorders impair learning, behavior, and language. They may cause a person to be sensitive to light or sound. Some developmental disorders

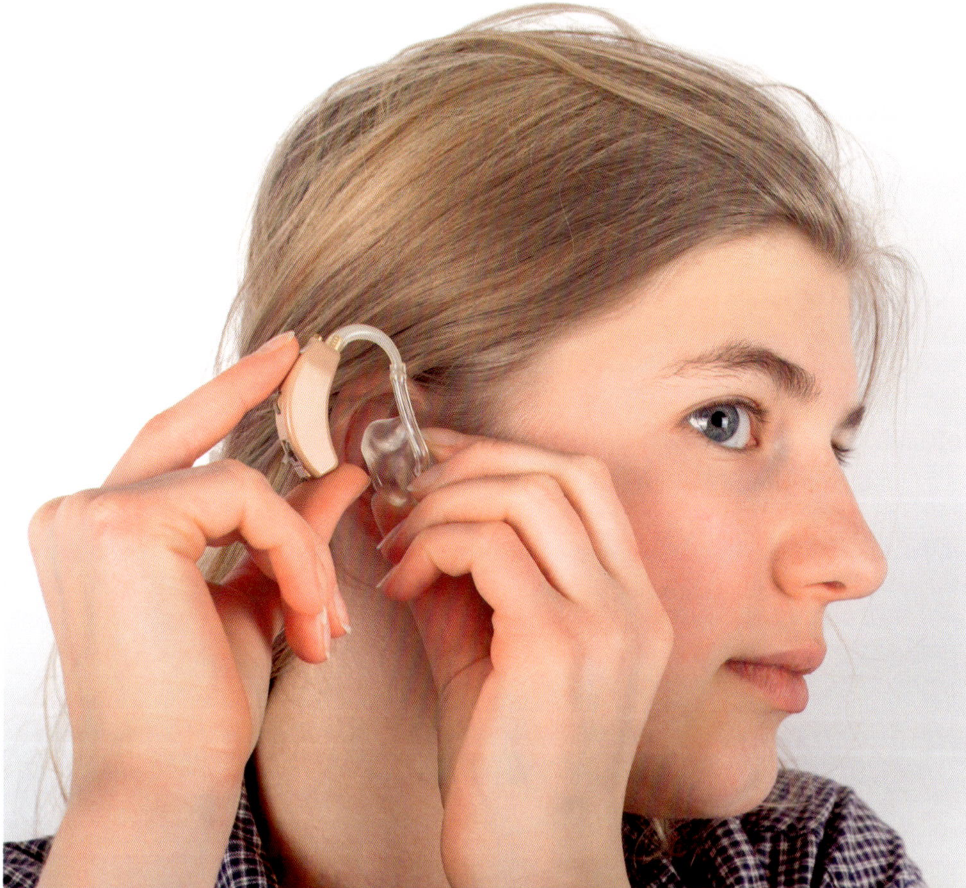

Hearing aids can help some forms of hearing loss caused by developmental disorders.

primarily affect the physical body. These include hearing loss and visual impairment.

Specific learning disorders (SLDs) are also developmental disorders. They can make it hard to read, write, or solve math problems. Other developmental disorders include intellectual disability (ID) and attention deficit **hyperactivity** disorder (ADHD). People with ID may find it difficult to learn school subjects and life skills. ADHD causes difficulties with paying attention and staying still. People with developmental disorders may face challenges throughout their lives. But as Greta's story shows, many can still lead rich lives.

CHAPTER ONE

THE HISTORY OF DEVELOPMENTAL DISORDERS

For much of history, people with developmental disorders have been abused. But those with ID have been treated particularly poorly. In ancient Rome, parents were told to abandon their children who had ID. The children were sometimes thrown in a river or left in the woods to die.

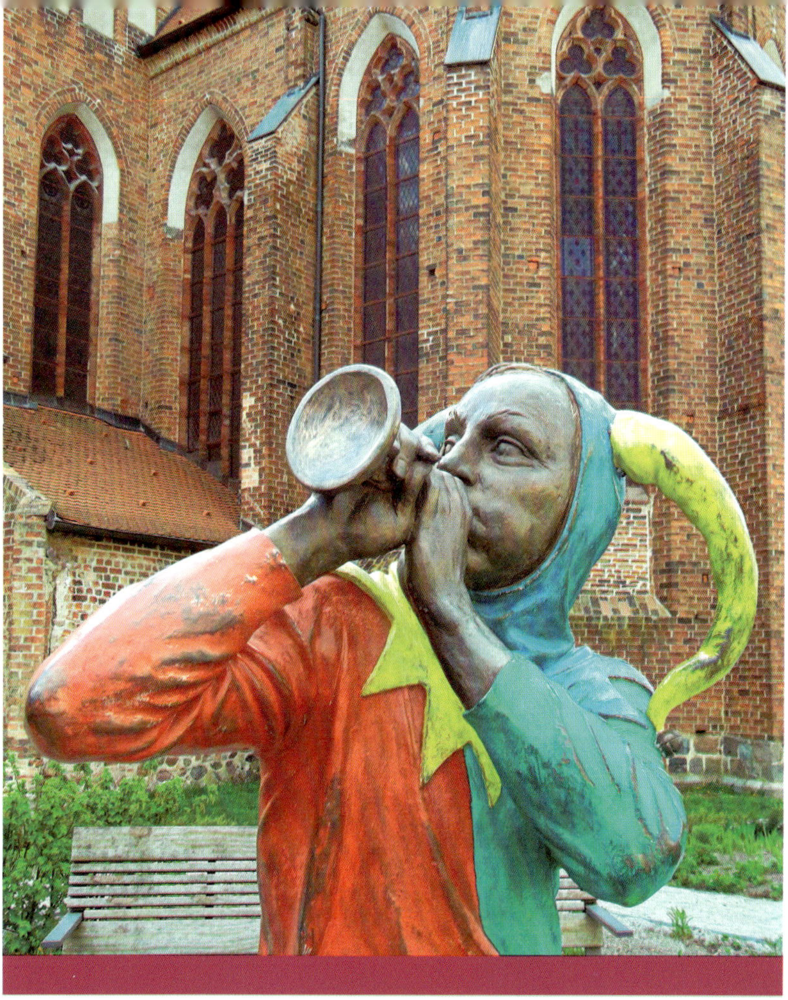

Court jesters entertained royals during the Middle Ages. Some jesters likely had intellectual disabilities.

In the Middle Ages, royal courts included fools. They provided entertainment. Some were likely people with ID, who were mocked and ridiculed by kings and queens.

FIGHTING FOR THEIR RIGHTS

In the following centuries, most people with ID were desperately poor. Some were confined to workhouses. These places provided shelter and work for those who were extremely poor. But living and working conditions were often harsh. Others with ID were driven out of their communities.

In the 1800s, reformers tried to help people with ID. One reformer was Samuel Gridley Howe. He set up a school in Massachusetts. Howe wanted people with ID to live full lives. At the school, students received basic education. They were

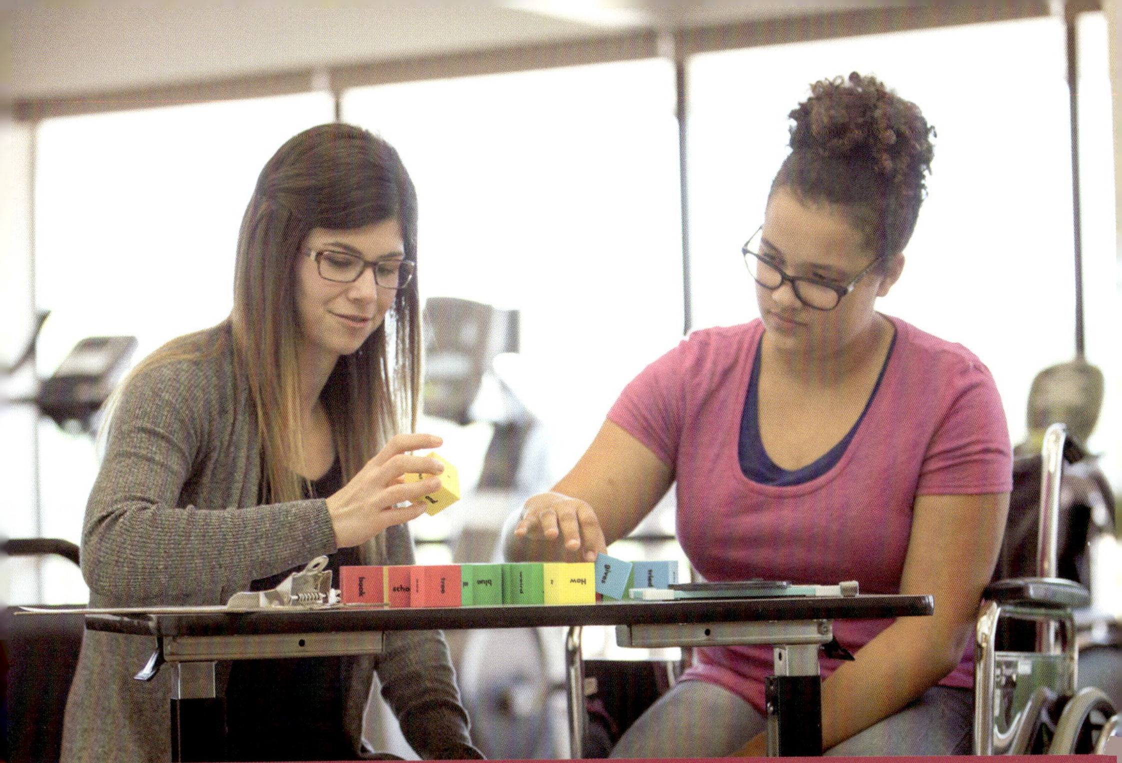

A therapist may help someone with skills like coordination. These skills help people with developmental disorders in their daily lives.

also taught job skills. When they left, they were prepared to work as farmhands or household help.

However, most people with ID were sent to overcrowded **institutions**. The living conditions were terrible. People received little to no treatment. Residents often spent their entire lives inside these buildings. They were ignored by their communities.

Life for the intellectually disabled was even worse in the early 1900s. Some scientists declared they were a threat to society. They did not want people with ID to have children. This is because ID can be passed from parent to child. Thousands of people with ID were **sterilized** against their will.

By the 1950s, parents who had children with ID fought to protect the rights of their children. Because of their work,

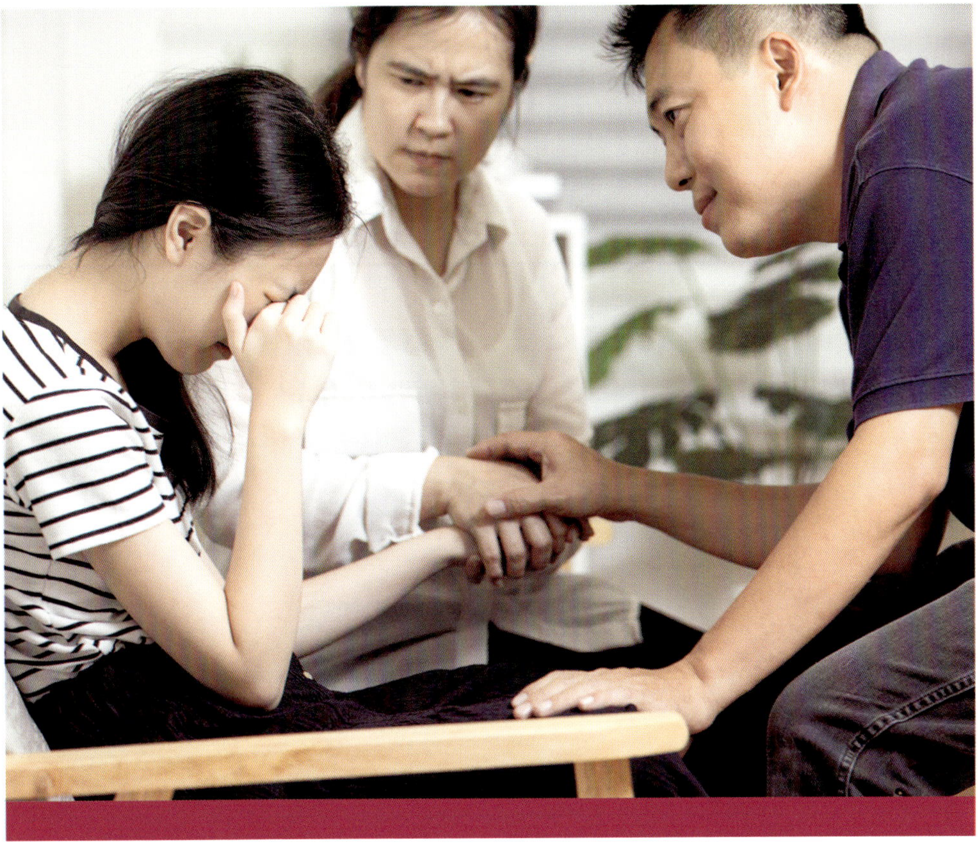

Family support is important to help someone cope with a developmental disorder.

many people with ID were able to leave institutions. In the decades that followed, children with ID were finally able to get a quality education. They began to get the care they needed.

ON THE SPECTRUM

In the past, some people with ASD were thought to be intellectually disabled. They were often treated cruelly. Many were sent to institutions. People with milder symptoms had an easier time fitting into society than those with more severe symptoms.

By the early 1900s, children with severe ASD were routinely put in mental hospitals. Medical experts thought nothing could help them. Doctors told parents to forget about their children.

In 1943, a doctor named Leo Kanner first defined autism. He thought only people

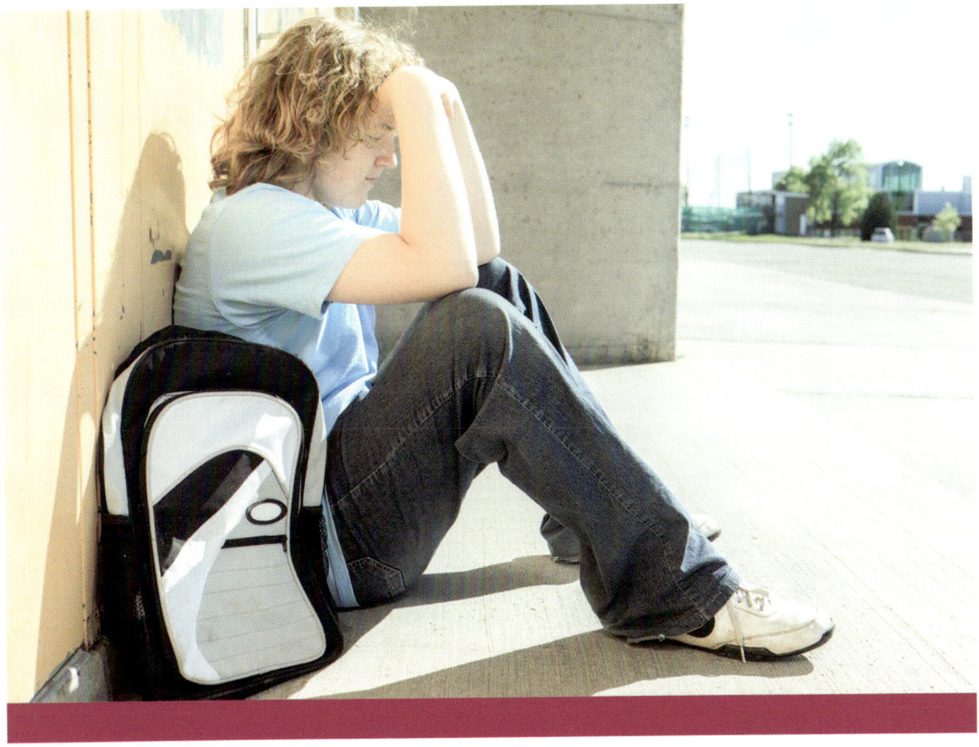

Someone with ASD may have a hard time fitting in with others.

with the worst symptoms were truly autistic. Doctors continued to learn more about the disorder. Later experts understood autism to include a wide range, or spectrum, of symptoms. That is why autism is now called autism spectrum disorder.

Bruno Bettelheim was a psychologist in the mid-1900s. He believed bad parenting caused autism. He singled out unemotional mothers for making their children autistic. His ideas were later proven wrong. But for years, parents felt terrible for causing their children's difficulties. Today, parents are far more hopeful because of new treatments to help people with ASD.

In the 1940s, Austrian doctor Hans Asperger defined a new condition. It later became known as Asperger's disorder. Children with the disorder displayed autism-like behavior. But they did not have other autism symptoms. For instance, they had average or high intelligence and had no trouble speaking. Asperger's is no longer considered a separate disorder. It is now thought to be a mild form of autism.

VICTOR, THE WILD BOY

Around 1800, a naked boy was found wandering in the woods of southern France. He couldn't speak. He rocked back and forth. He hated to be touched. Today, he probably would be diagnosed with ASD.

A doctor named Jean-Marc-Gaspard Itard named him Victor. For five years, Itard tried to teach Victor to speak. He had little success. But his effort was an early example of special education for a child with ASD.

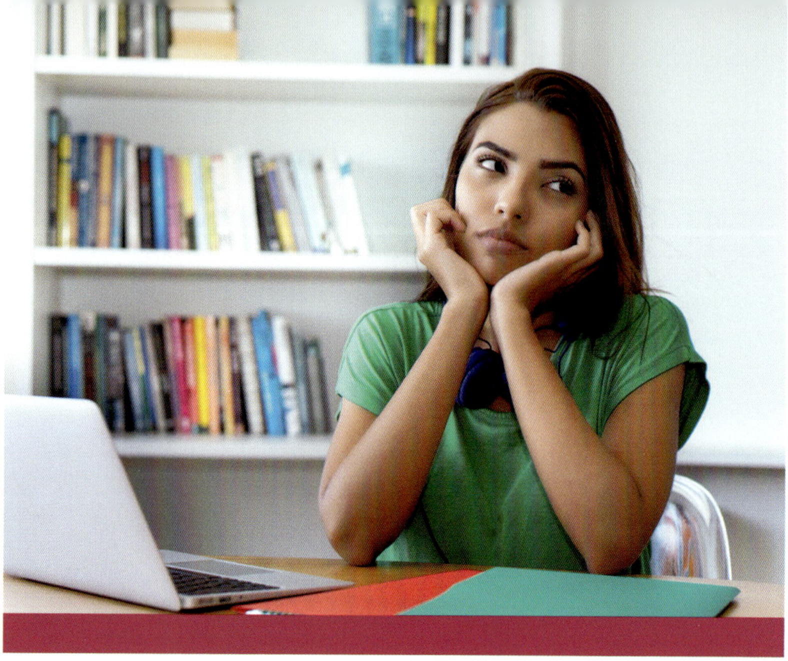

ADHD can make it difficult to concentrate on schoolwork.

PAYING ATTENTION

There have always been people who have trouble paying attention or staying still. But severe cases were not called a disorder until 1798. Scottish doctor Sir Alexander Crichton studied people with these problems all over Europe. He wrote about people who could not focus on “any one object." They were easily distracted by even "a slight noise." Heat, cold, or light could "destroy constant attention."[2] Crichton's observations were perhaps the first written description of ADHD.

Many years would pass before there was an effective treatment for ADHD. American doctor Charles Bradley worked with children with behavior problems in the 1930s. Today, experts believe these children would be diagnosed with ADHD. He performed medical tests to study the brains of these children. But the tests often resulted in headaches. Bradley offered them a drug called Benzedrine for the pain. The **stimulant** did not make their headaches go away. But it did improve their attention. Benzedrine is no longer given to people with ADHD. But other stimulants are.

In 1968, the American Psychiatric Association (APA) named the disorder. The APA called it hyperkinetic reaction of childhood. It was renamed in 1980 as attention deficit disorder (ADD). There were two types of ADD. In one type, people displayed hyperactivity. In the other type, people experienced more difficulties with attention. The diagnosis changed again in

1987. The disorder was renamed ADHD. ADHD is grouped into three presentations. There is a hyperactive-impulsive presentation and an inattentive presentation. Patients who show both types of symptoms have a combined presentation.

FIDGETY PHIL

German doctor Heinrich Hoffman was an expert in mental disorders. In 1844, he wrote a children's book. One character was Fidgety Phil. Phil's father was sick of Phil's fidgeting. He wanted him to sit still at the dinner table. Phil ignored him. Soon his chair fell over. The table crashed to the floor, ruining dinner. Hoffman possibly based Phil on patients with ADHD.

CHAPTER TWO

NOTABLE DEVELOPMENTAL DISORDERS

Developmental disorders have various symptoms. People often first display symptoms when they are children. But sometimes, people do not receive a diagnosis until they are teens or adults.

Intellectual disability affects about 1 percent of the population. People with ID

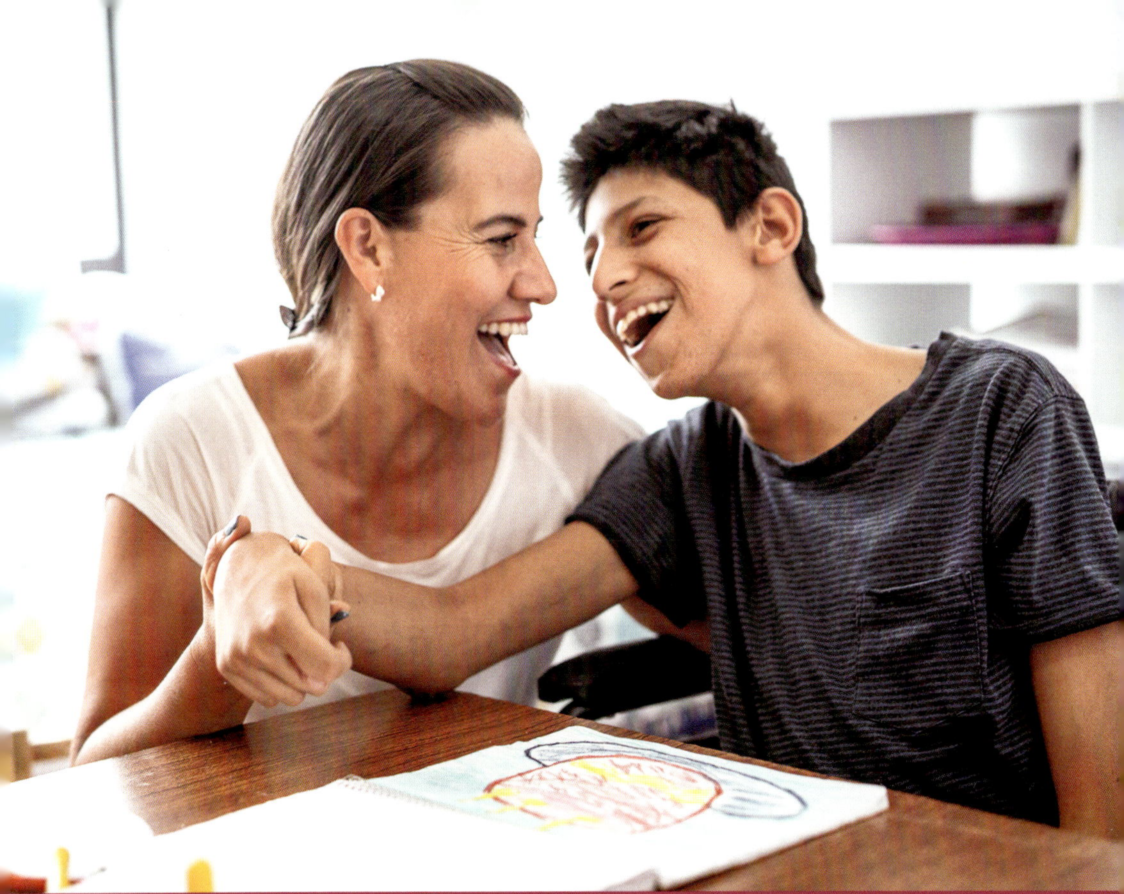

Someone with ID may need additional care from a parent or guardian.

struggle with learning and solving problems. They also have limited social skills. Everyday tasks can be difficult. They may need help washing, dressing, or organizing their days. Children with ID may walk and talk later than other children. They may also have trouble understanding rules.

Intelligence quotient (IQ) tests are used to diagnose ID. IQ tests determine a person's ability to learn new things. They also test memory and problem-solving skills. A score of 70 or less on an IQ test can be a sign of ID. Other tests that measure a person's ability to perform everyday skills are also used for diagnosis.

CHALLENGES WITH COMMUNICATING

People with ASD find it difficult to socialize with others. They may have trouble speaking. They may struggle to

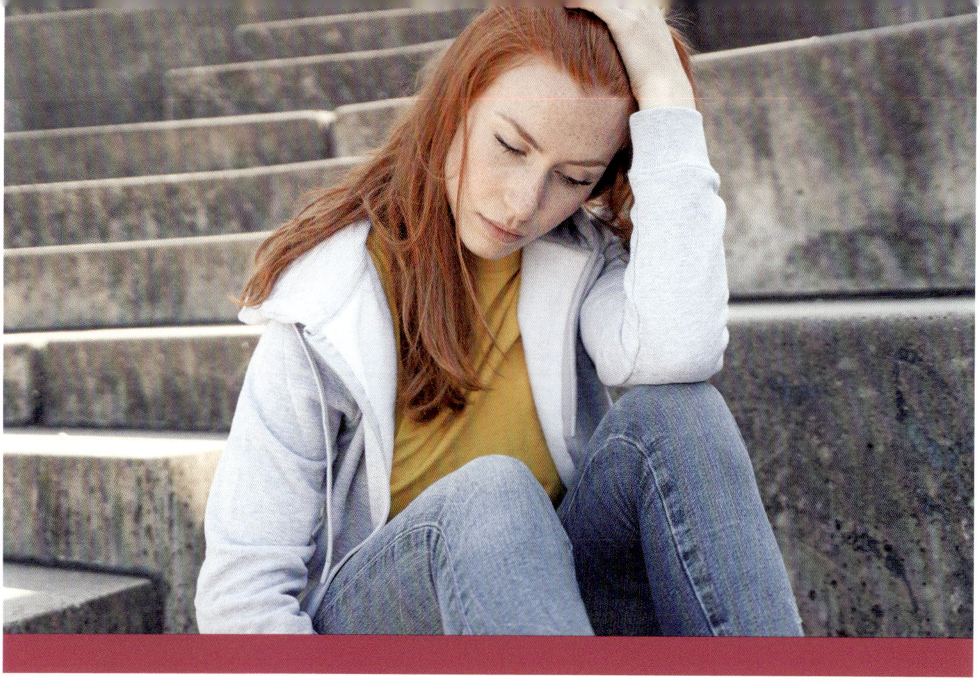

Someone with ASD may find social interactions challenging.

understand nonverbal communication. For instance, they may not know how to read other people's facial expressions or body languagc. Symptoms range from mild to severe.

People with ASD often avoid eye contact and express little interest in others. Sometimes, they repeat phrases other

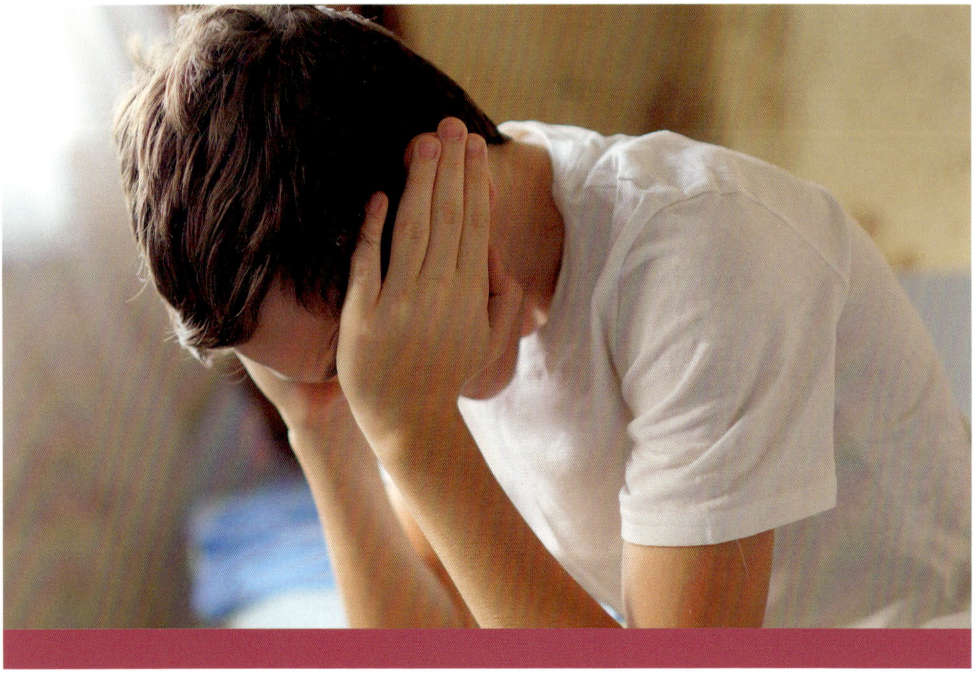

ASD may cause someone to be sensitive to noises.

people have said. They may make repetitive movements, such as rocking back and forth or flapping their hands. Many do not like to be touched. They may also be very sensitive to noises, smells, and tastes.

Autism symptoms usually appear by age two or three. Early signs include a child not smiling and not responding to his or her name. A medical professional diagnoses ASD after observing how a child talks and acts.

About one in fifty-four US children has ASD. It is about four times more common in boys than girls. ASD symptoms in girls may be harder to spot. Girls may be diagnosed less often as a result. Researchers also think that girls may have **genes** that protect them from ASD. There are many genes that are related to ASD. On average, girls have more autism-related changes in their genes when showing symptoms than boys do.

It is not uncommon for people with mild symptoms to learn they are autistic in their teens or later. Sometimes, the diagnosis is a relief. A woman named Alanna Whitney spoke to the *Washington Post* about hers.

AUTISM AND VACCINES

In 1998, a British doctor linked vaccines with autism. His study was done incorrectly. He ignored data that didn't fit with his ideas. He lost the right to practice medicine. But it led some people to falsely believe that children can get autism from vaccines. The Centers for Disease Control and Prevention (CDC) has studied the issue. The CDC and many other scientific organizations found no evidence that vaccines cause autism. Childhood vaccines are very safe. They protect children from serious diseases.

“It was the answer to every question I’d ever had,” she said. “It was kind of like a go-ahead to . . . embrace myself for who I am.”[3]

A LACK OF FOCUS

ADHD is one of the most common developmental disorders. About 8.4 percent of children have ADHD. About 2.5 percent of adults have this disorder.

Research shows brain differences between people with ADHD and people without ADHD. The brain is made of many parts. These parts communicate with each other. The way these parts interact may be different in people with ADHD. This can affect focus and attention. Other studies show that people with ADHD have a smaller frontal lobe. This region is located in the front of the brain. It is responsible for memory, impulse control, and planning.

People with ADHD may also have different levels of brain chemicals called neurotransmitters. One example is dopamine. It is related to motivation. Another neurotransmitter is called norepinephrine. It can help with attention. Levels of these chemicals may be lower in people with ADHD.

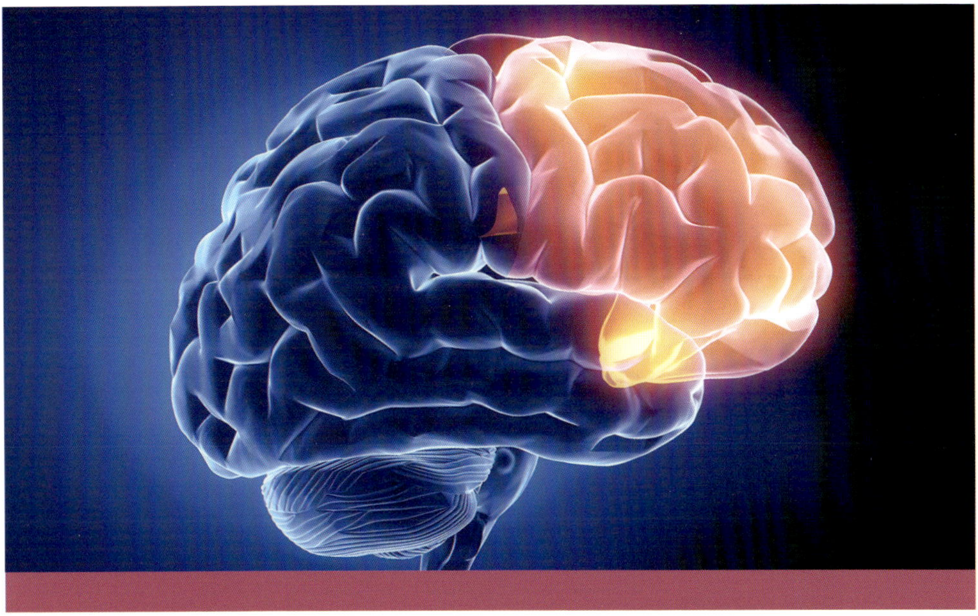

The frontal lobe is one region of the brain that is responsible for impulse control and decision-making.

People with ADHD often find it hard to pay attention to anything for long. They have trouble focusing on tasks and following instructions. They may also squirm and fidget at their desks. Another symptom of ADHD is being impulsive. People with this disorder sometimes make rushed decisions and engage in risky behavior. These symptoms can cause serious trouble at home and in school.

ADHD has long been thought to be more common in boys than girls. But some experts believe girls may be underdiagnosed. The reason may be that symptoms in girls can be different. Boys with ADHD are often overactive and disruptive. Girls with the disorder tend to be unfocused and forgetful.

People with ADHD usually have symptoms before the age of twelve. Specialists in ADHD diagnose the disorder.

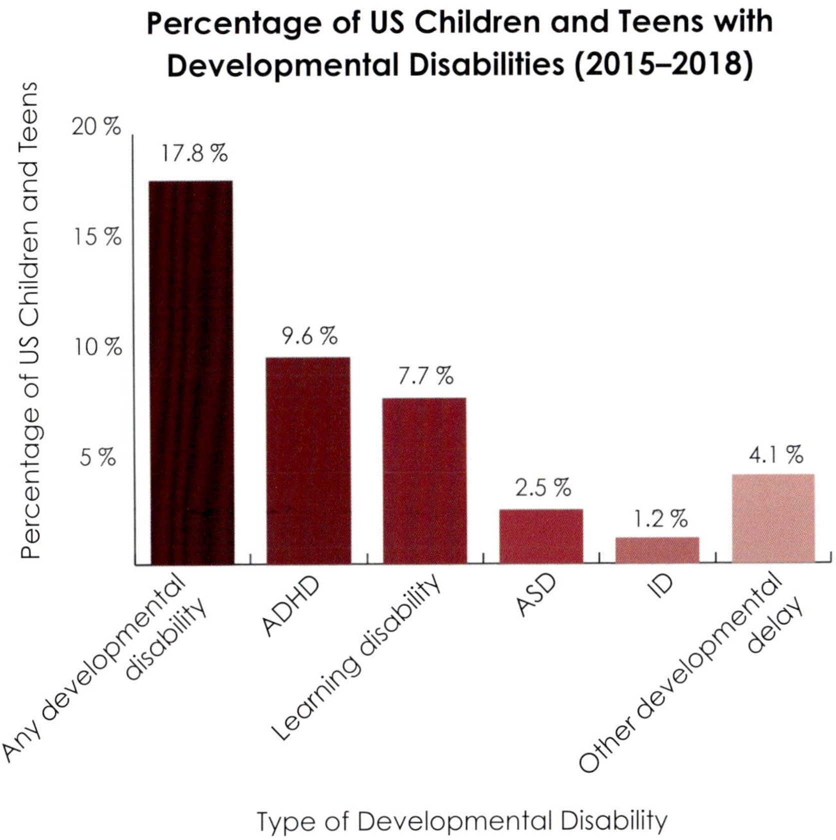

Source: Benjamin Zablotsky, PhD, and Lindsey I. Black, MPH, "Prevalence of Children Aged 3–17 Years with Developmental Disabilities, by Urbanicity: United States, 2015–2018." National Health Statistics Reports, *February 19, 2020, p. 3.*

The US Department of Health and Human Services collects data on children and teens with developmental disabilities. A person can have more than one type of developmental disability.

They gather information by talking to a child's parents and teachers. An ADHD diagnosis is made from observations. Sometimes this can lead to the wrong diagnosis. For example, a parent or teacher may report that a child's behavior is more extreme than it actually is. Psychological tests can help rule out other conditions that

TIC DISORDERS

Some children develop tics. These are sudden sounds or movements that are made over and over again. Tics may cause people to shake their heads repeatedly. They may feel the need to keep clearing their throats. Other people may have a hard time understanding the behaviors of someone with a tic disorder. This can make it difficult for children with a tic disorder to make friends.

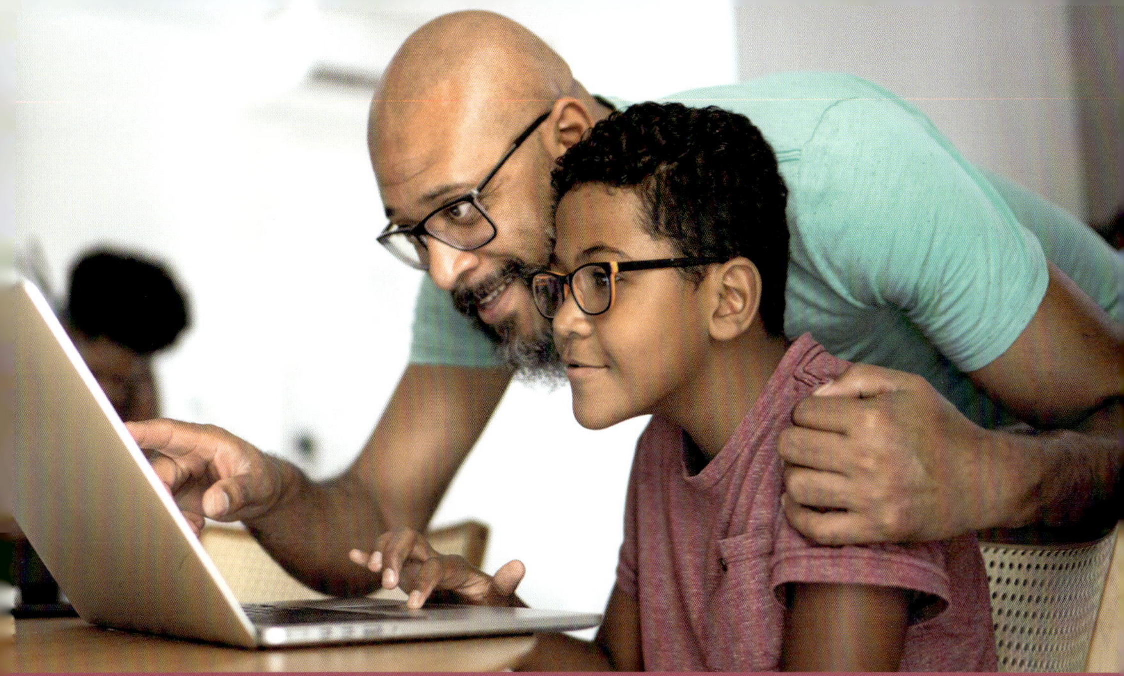

Family members may share a developmental disorder such as ADHD. They may be able to offer advice on how to cope with the disorder.

have similar symptoms to ADHD. These include anxiety, depression, and ASD.

Terry Matlen is an ADHD therapist who herself has ADHD. She describes the disorder as "a **chronic** sense of [being] overwhelmed." That can create a feeling of defeat and failure. She encourages others with ADHD. "You're not broken. You're not helpless," she reminds them. "You just need a little extra help."[4]

CAUSES OF DEVELOPMENTAL DISORDERS

Often, a mix of factors lead to a developmental disorder. One is genetics. Parents may have genes related to ADHD. Children may inherit these genes from their parents. A parent with ADHD is likely to have a child with the same condition.

Developmental disorders may develop during pregnancy. A pregnant mother may have an infection. This can affect her baby's development. Alcohol use during pregnancy can cause fetal alcohol syndrome (FAS). Children with FAS may struggle with memory. They may also develop ID. Premature birth or a low birth weight are other risk factors. A child's exposure to lead and other **toxins** are other possible causes.

CEREBRAL PALSY

Cerebral palsy (CP) can be a serious developmental disorder. It affects a person's movement. About one in every 345 children in the United States has CP. CP is usually caused by abnormal brain development in babies. But it can also be caused by certain infections or head injuries. People with CP cannot control their muscles properly. They might have problems maintaining balance. Symptoms vary from person to person. They can be mild or severe.

CHAPTER THREE

DEVELOPMENTAL DISORDERS AND EVERYDAY LIFE

Developmental disorders can make daily life difficult. People with these disorders may struggle at home, at school, and at work. Because of these challenges, some may find it difficult to reach their full potential. But many people learn to cope with their symptoms over time.

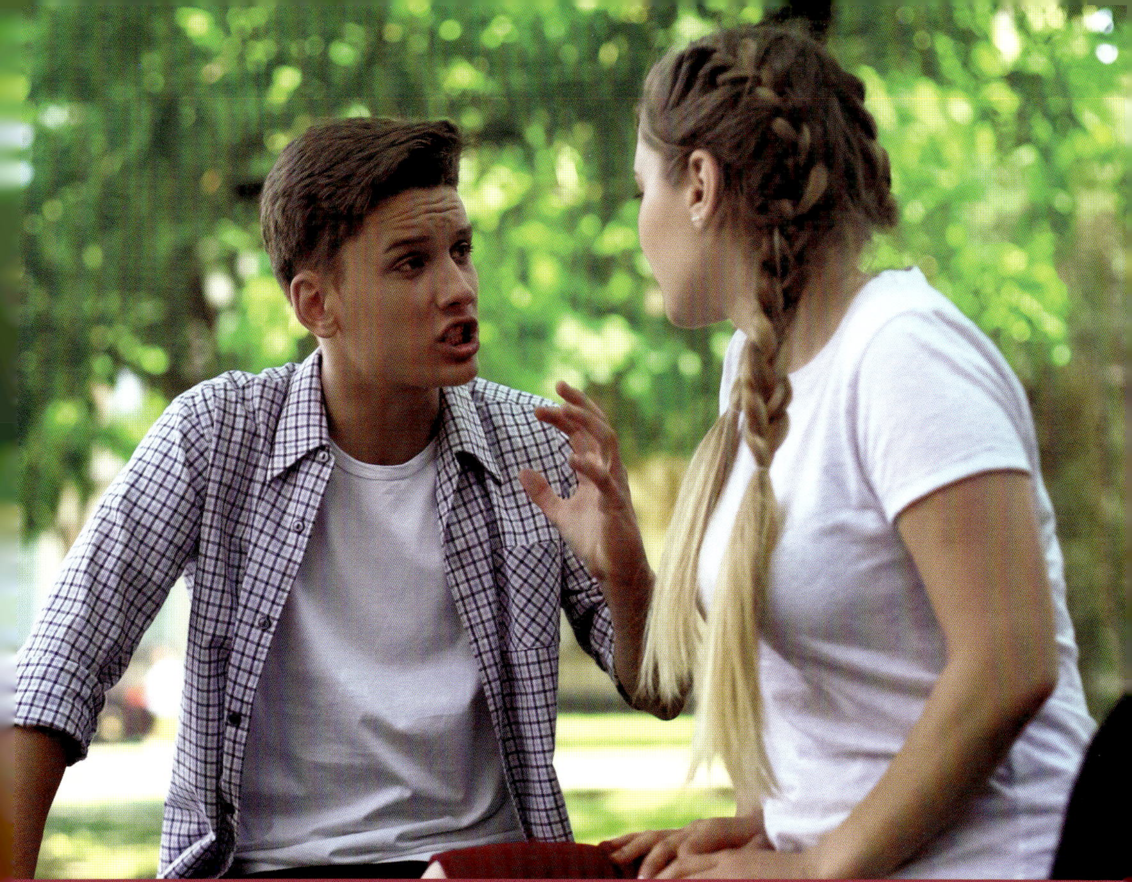

Someone with a developmental disorder may get overwhelmed or frustrated easily.

DEALING WITH ID

Approximately 85 percent of people with intellectual disabilities have mild symptoms. But they may still have a hard time performing everyday tasks. They often

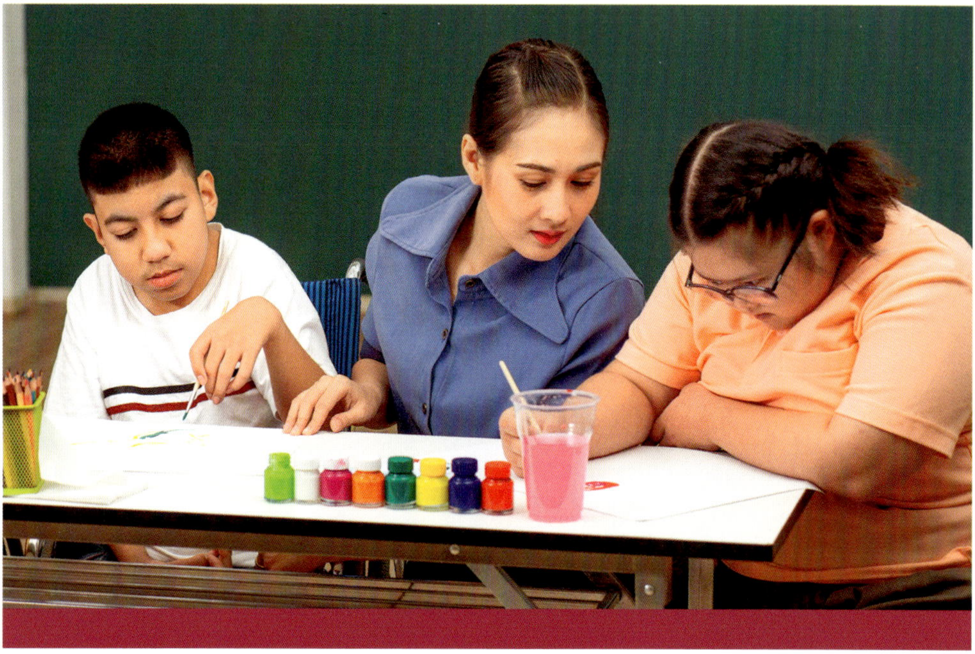

People with developmental disorders may take special education classes.

have trouble taking care of themselves. For instance, they may need help getting dressed and making meals. People with ID can also have problems interacting with others. They may have difficulties expressing themselves. They may struggle to understand others. As a result, their relationships with friends and family can suffer.

At school, people with ID have a harder time learning than other students do. As they fall behind, they often become frustrated. They may act out or get depressed. This type of stress is particularly difficult for teens.

Life for people with severe symptoms is even harder. Sometimes, they can barely communicate with others. In severe cases, people with ID may have to receive special care. They may be unable to live independently.

ASD CHALLENGES

People with ASD have trouble communicating with others. This problem affects their lives in many ways. They may have a hard time making friends. They may find it difficult to share their emotions or understand other people's feelings. They may not react in a way others expect. For example, a person with autism may not look excited when he hears good news. Or he may react strongly and scream when he is frustrated. Because of these problems, about 40 percent of children with ASD spend little time with friends. They may

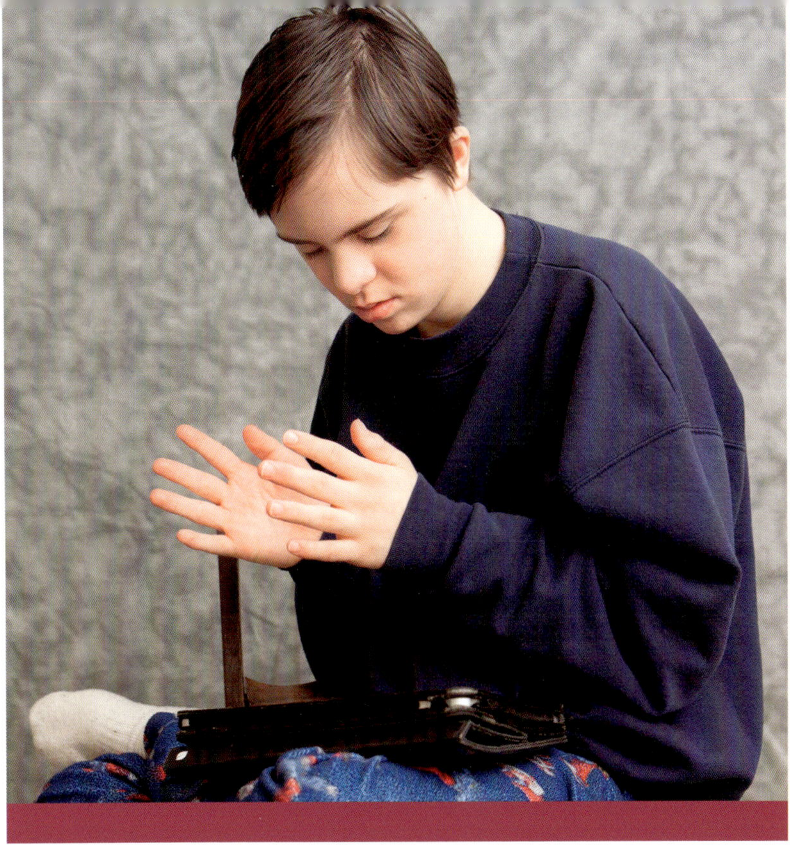

A tablet can be a useful communication device for someone with ASD.

also struggle to maintain relationships with their relatives.

Bullies also sometimes target people with ASD. Bullying expert Catherine Bradshaw explained the problem. “Children with autism spectrum disorder aren’t very good at picking up on things like sarcasm and humor," she said. "They can be . . . made fun of in front of groups and not understand it."[5]

To deal with others, people with ASD sometimes resort to carefully controlling their behavior. They force themselves to make eye contact. They monitor their facial expressions. They speak in rehearsed responses. But these efforts to please others can be exhausting. They may cause a person with ASD to feel depressed.

Many people with ASD are of average or even high intelligence. But their disorder makes it hard for them to succeed in school. Students with ASD often do not understand what their teachers expect from them.

ASD AND MASKS

Wearing masks was required in many places during the COVID-19 pandemic. This helped prevent the spread of the disease. But wearing masks was difficult for some people with ASD. They are often very sensitive to touch. They may dislike the feeling of the mask and ear straps.

The company Rafi Nova came up with a solution. It made a soft mask for people with ASD. Its straps connected behind the head. It also lifted away from the mouth, making breathing easier.

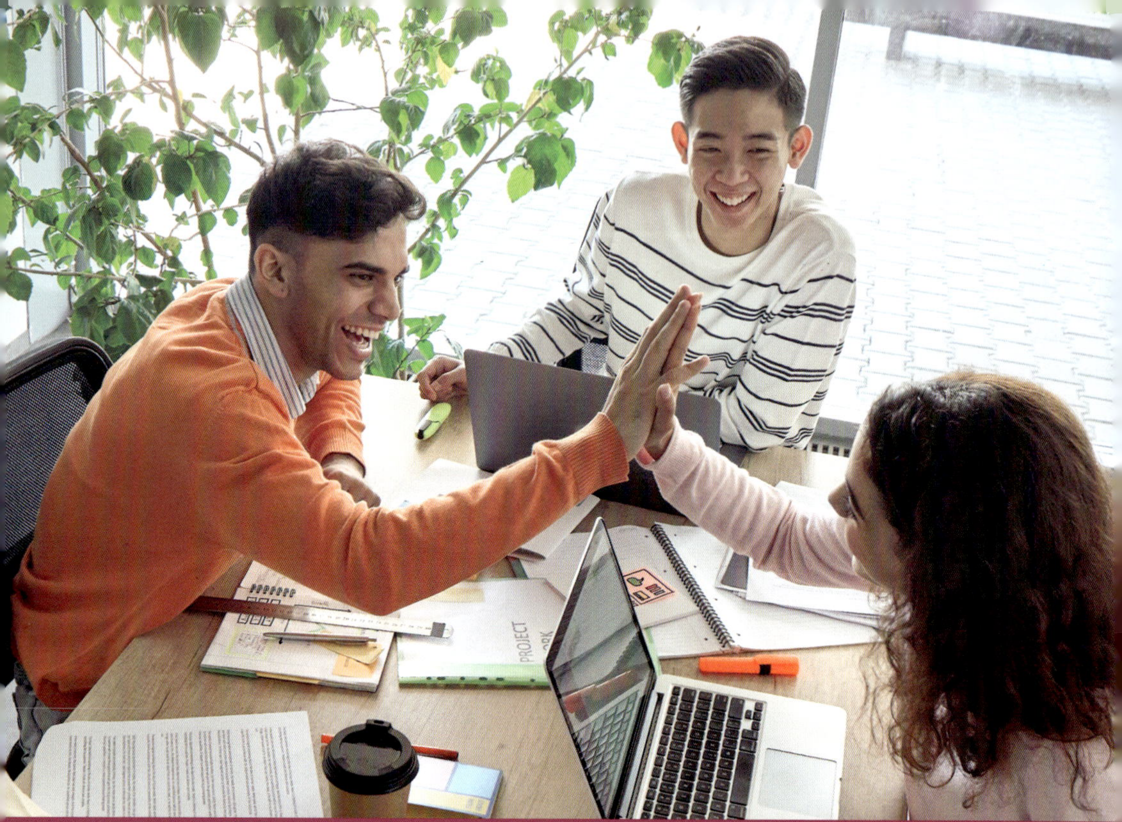

Creative problem-solving can be a valuable skill in the workplace.

As adults, people with autism often struggle in the workplace. They may have trouble dealing with coworkers and bosses. They may have trouble finding work at all. For emotional and financial reasons, many cannot live independently.

But recently some companies have started recruiting people with ASD. They recognize that these people have special skills and talents. Many are highly focused. They may pay very close attention to detail. They also may have excellent memories. The ability to think differently and creatively is valuable. They may come up with new solutions to old problems.

LIVING WITH ADHD

At every stage of life, coping with ADHD can be hard. Children and teens struggle in school. They often cannot focus on lessons or follow teachers' instructions. Sometimes they are punished for behaviors they cannot control. Students with ADHD are likely to talk too much in class. They may also interrupt their teachers. They find it difficult to wait in line and take turns.

As adults, people with ADHD have a hard time with everyday tasks. They often do not organize their time well. At work, they may miss deadlines and forget meetings. Their lack of impulse control can also get them into trouble. They may make hasty financial decisions or abuse alcohol and drugs.

People with ADHD sometimes blame themselves for their problems. This can lead

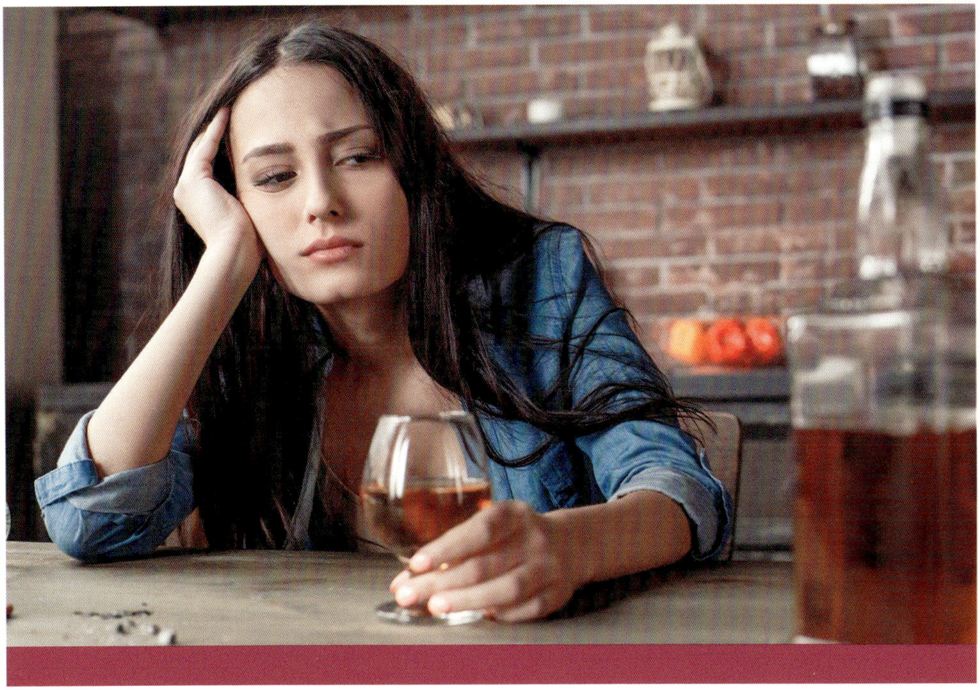

Alcohol use can worsen symptoms of ADHD.

to low self-esteem. Dealing with ADHD can be frustrating. It can leave people feeling depressed, anxious, and stressed.

Schools can help students with ADHD succeed. Teachers can give these students more time on tests. They can praise good work so students feel confident. Technology

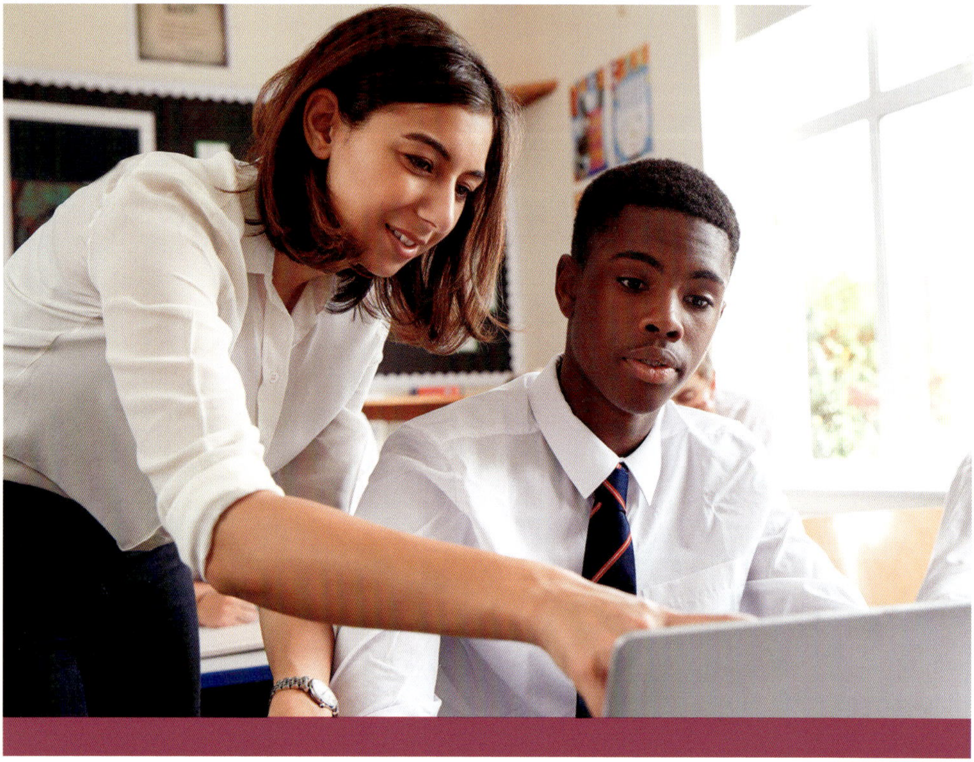

A teacher can create a learning environment that helps students with ADHD find success.

can also help. For example, computers with audio can aid reading. Students can hear the words as they read. That can help them follow the text better.

Workplaces can also help people with ADHD do their best. People with ADHD may be distracted by noises. They can ask to wear earphones at work. They can also request desks in quiet corners. Bright lights can also bother people with ADHD. Employers can change the lights or bulbs to help.

FAMOUS PEOPLE WITH ADHD

Having ADHD can be frustrating. But by managing this disorder, many people with ADHD have successful careers. Justin Timberlake became a famous singer. Tim Howard emerged as a world-class soccer champ. Emma Watson starred in the *Harry Potter* movie franchise. Dave Grohl played in the bands Nirvana and Foo Fighters.

CHAPTER FOUR

TREATING DEVELOPMENTAL DISORDERS

People with developmental disorders face numerous challenges. But many have found hope through treatment. People with developmental disorders can learn to cope with their symptoms. Many are able to live independent lives. Other people with developmental disorders may need

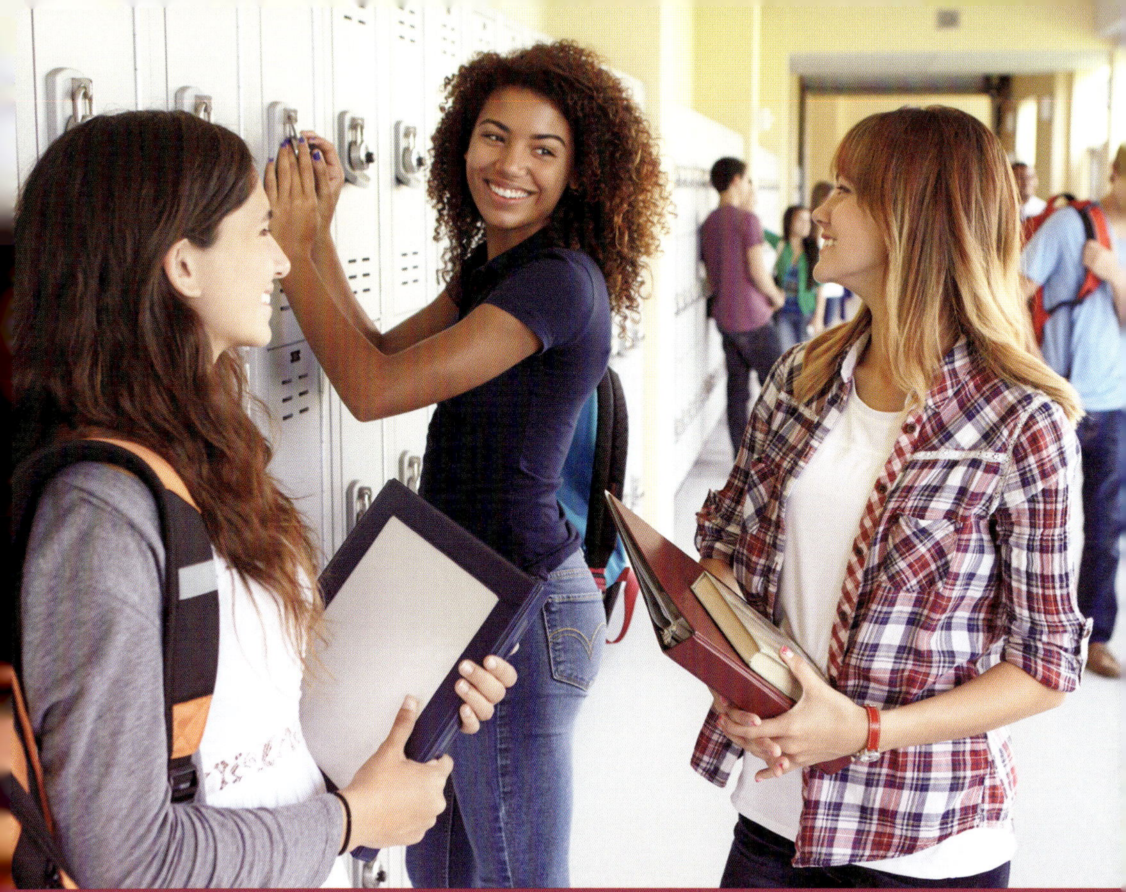

Many people with developmental disorders learn to manage their symptoms.

additional care. They are still able to have full, happy lives. Many learn to manage their disorders with treatment. They learn skills that help them in daily life. They are able to lead successful, satisfying lives.

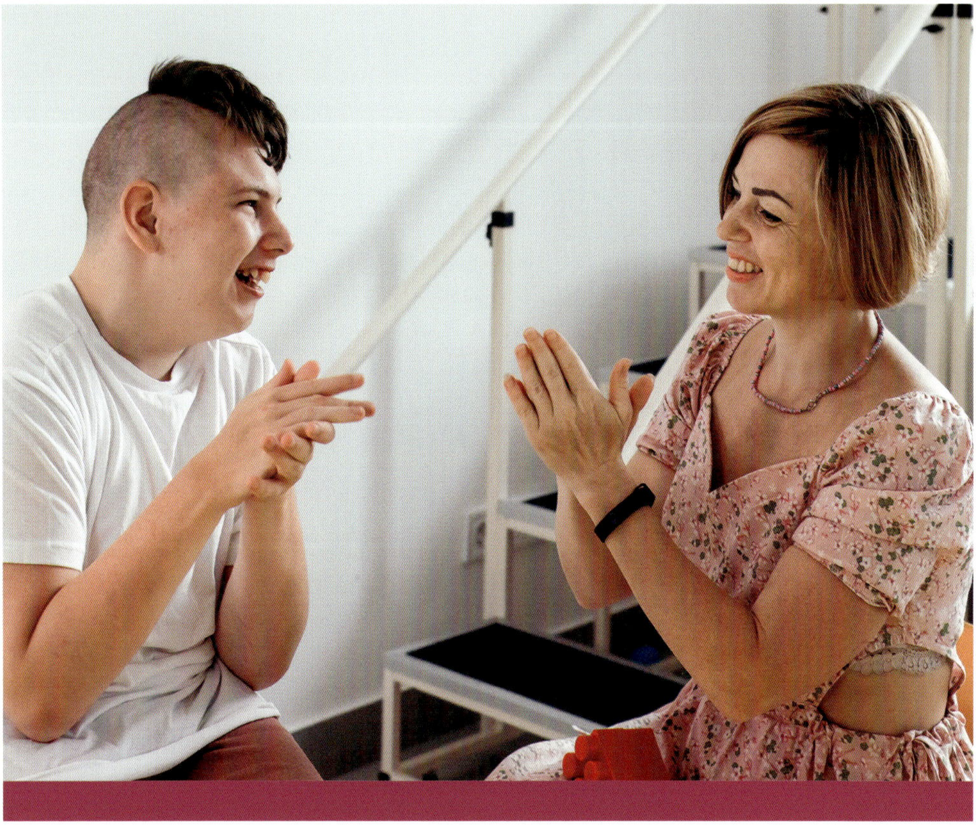

A therapist may work with a child with ID on behavioral skills.

BECOMING INDEPENDENT

People with severe ID need help to take care of their daily needs. But people with mild symptoms can develop social and life skills. These skills can help them live fairly independent lives.

Early diagnosis can make a big difference. Specialists can help babies and toddlers learn helpful skills. They work with the children's family to make plans that best fit the children's needs.

At school, children with ID attend special education classes. Trained teachers create lessons specially designed for each student. They teach subjects like reading and math. They also teach social skills so students can get along with others. Students learn practical skills so they can take better care of themselves.

Students with ID can also learn how to properly do a job. This training will help them become more independent as adults. Family members often provide additional emotional and financial support. This helps adults with ID live successful lives.

THERAPY FOR ASD

People with ASD can learn social skills and behaviors to help them cope. The earlier this therapy begins, the better. Children can be taught ways to deal with autism. They can use these skills for the rest of their lives.

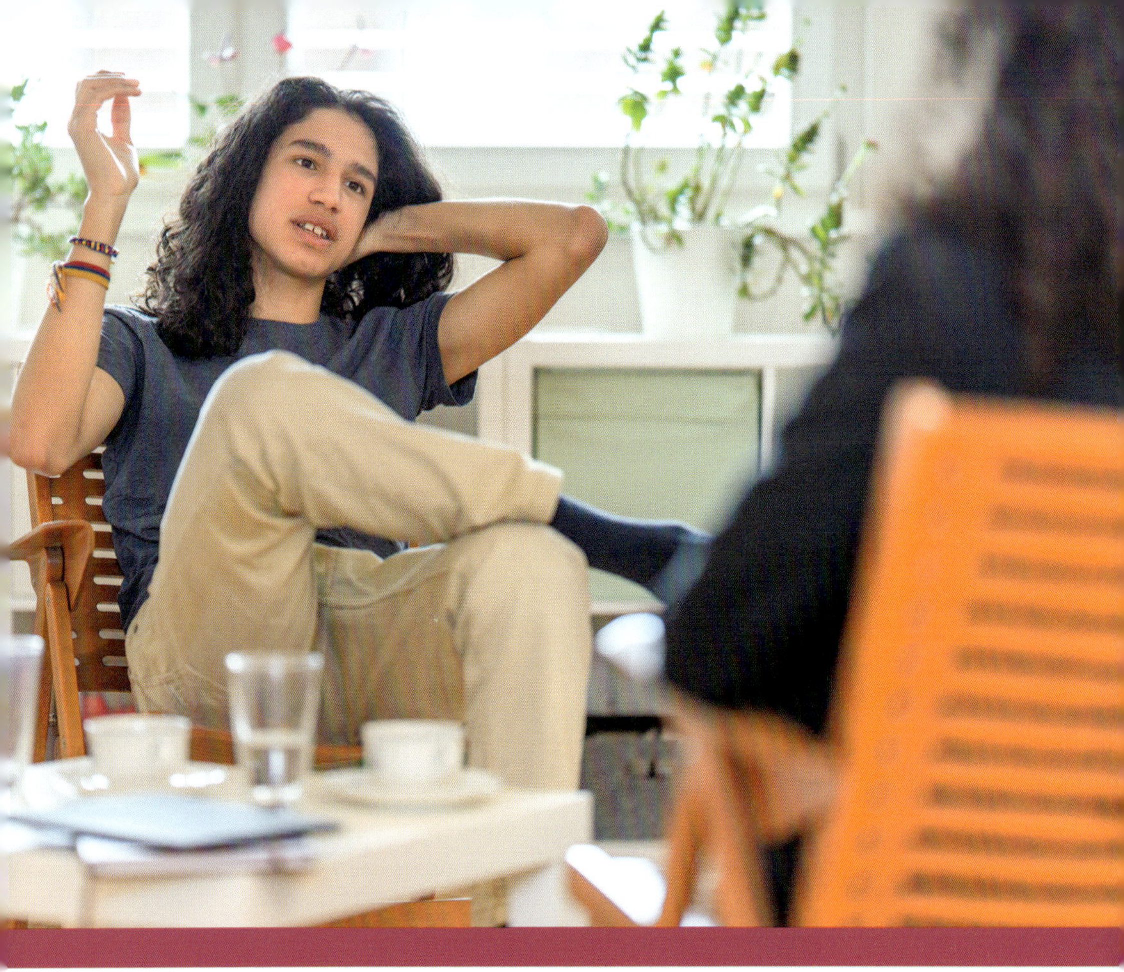

A teen with ASD may speak with a therapist about symptoms.

One popular therapy is called applied behavior analysis. Therapists use it to teach skills to people with ASD. The lessons vary with each person's needs. For instance, people may be taught to make eye contact. A therapist breaks down the desired behavior into small steps. When people with ASD complete a step, they get a reward. This makes them want to repeat the behavior.

Some people with ASD benefit from occupational therapy. It teaches them skills such as bathing and dressing. This therapy can help people with ASD live more independently. People with ASD may have difficulty with movement. They can receive physical therapy to improve their balance and coordination. They may work with a speech therapist if they have difficulty communicating. In addition, many students with ASD attend special education classes.

FINDING A VOICE ONLINE

In 2019, the *New York Times* published an award-winning editorial by Asaka Park. She describes her life as a teen with ASD:

> *I'm keenly attuned to the unwritten rules of social interaction. . . . While I easily grasp abstract concepts, I often can't convert them into . . . step-by-step actions, making it difficult to communicate gracefully. . . . On social media though, I'm a completely different person. I'm dynamic. I'm assertive. I'm people-oriented.*

Asaka Park, "I'm a Disabled Teenager, and Social Media Is My Lifeline," New York Times, *June 5, 2019. www.nytimes.com*

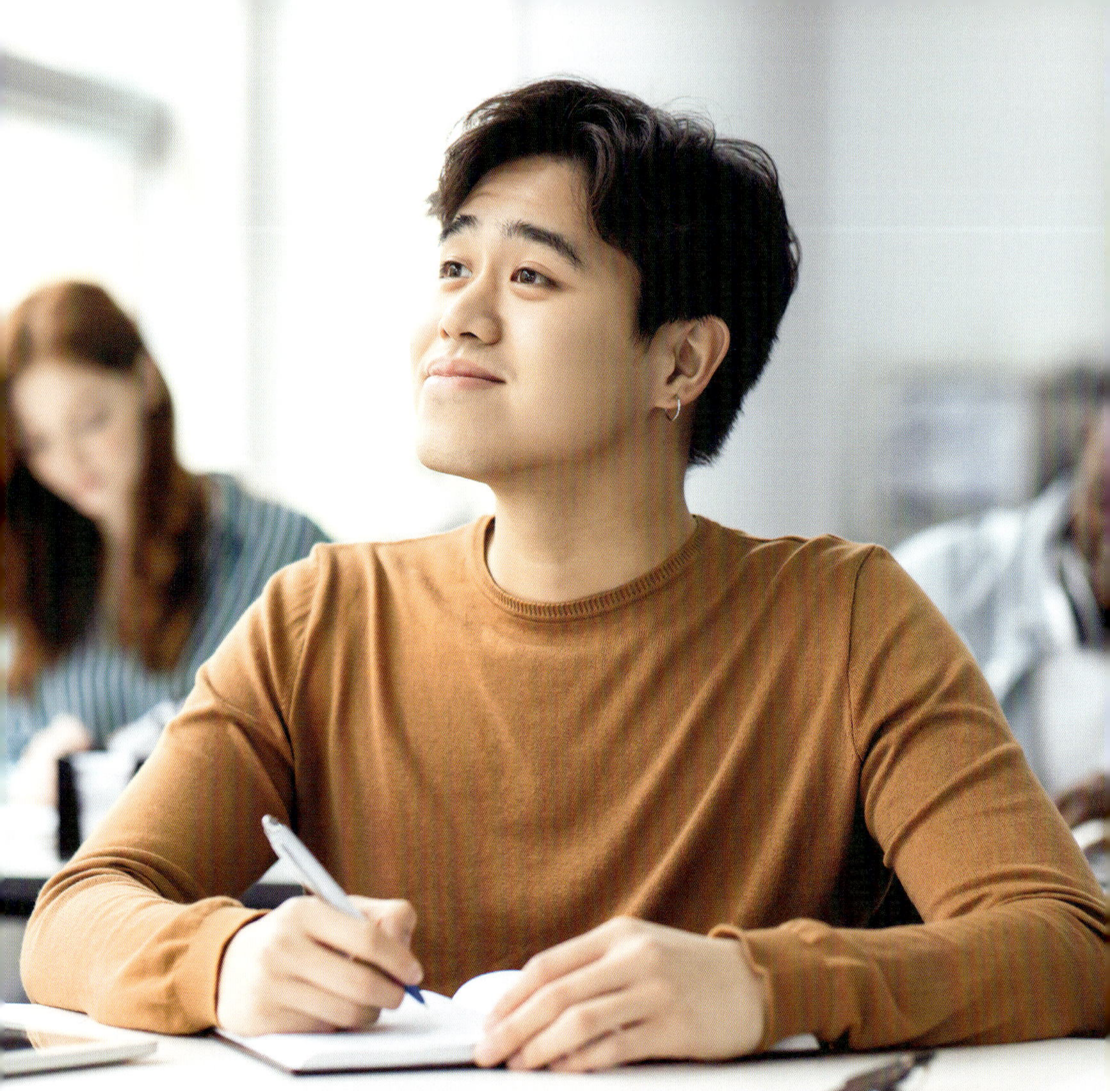

Keeping track of assignments in a planner can help a student with ADHD remember his work.

ADHD RELIEF

ADHD can be treated with medication.

Stimulants such as Ritalin can relieve ADHD

symptoms. Stimulants increase levels of dopamine in the brain. These medications do have some side effects, though. They might make people irritable or raise their heart rate and blood pressure.

Many people with ADHD combine medication with therapy. Behavioral therapists teach them how to behave in social settings. Therapists talk with their patients about their problems. Therapists help patients deal with past failures.

People with ADHD can do much to relieve symptoms on their own. They can establish a routine to keep themselves

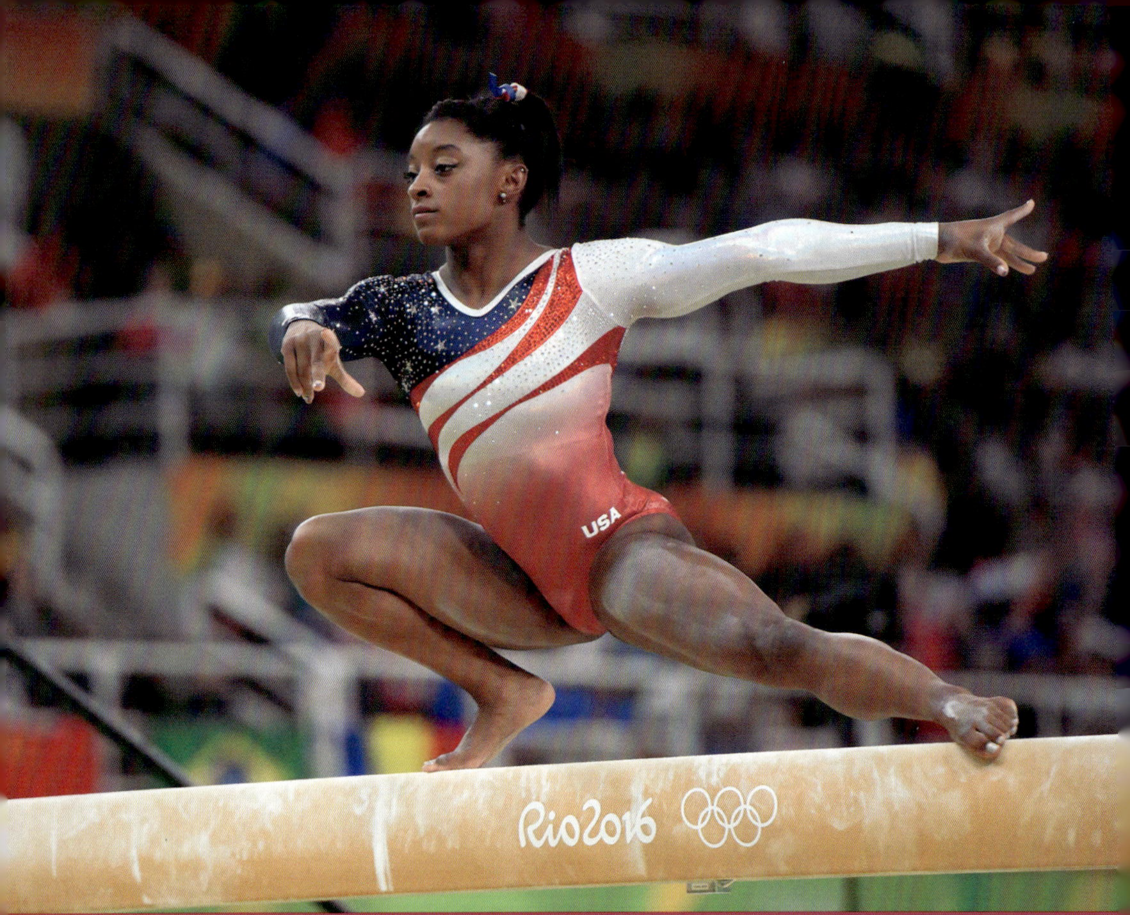

Celebrities, including Simone Biles, have spoken about their neurodiversity.

from getting overwhelmed. They can write down appointments so they do not forget them. They can also create to-do lists. They may break tasks down into small, easy-to-finish actions.

Some teens with ADHD find solace in sports. The disorder may help them stay alert and active on a busy playing field. Champion swimmer Michael Phelps has ADHD. So does Olympic gymnast Simone Biles. When her disorder made news, Biles did not mind. “Having ADHD . . . is nothing to be ashamed of,” she tweeted.[6]

NEURODIVERSITY

Current treatments have helped many people with developmental disorders. But recently some of these people have questioned the goal of some treatments. They are not sure they want to be trained to think and act like others. They may not see themselves as having a disorder at all. Instead, they believe their way of thinking is natural. It is just different from that of other people.

This idea is called neurodiversity. The word was invented in the 1990s by researcher Judy Singer. Singer herself has autism. She thinks it is good that people think in different ways. Autistic writer John Elder Robison also embraces neurodiversity. He has said, "Society needs the exceptional thinkers that the neurodiversity world produces."[7]

Neurodiversity activists have banded together on social media. They want to see changes in schools. They think special education teachers should make the most of their students' strengths. For instance, teachers could encourage students with

SAVANT SYNDROME

People with savant syndrome have great mental skills in a very limited area. Some people with savant syndrome can do complex math problems in their heads. Others can play a piece of music after hearing it only once. Some people with savant syndrome can easily memorize entire books. Half of the people with savant syndrome have ASD.

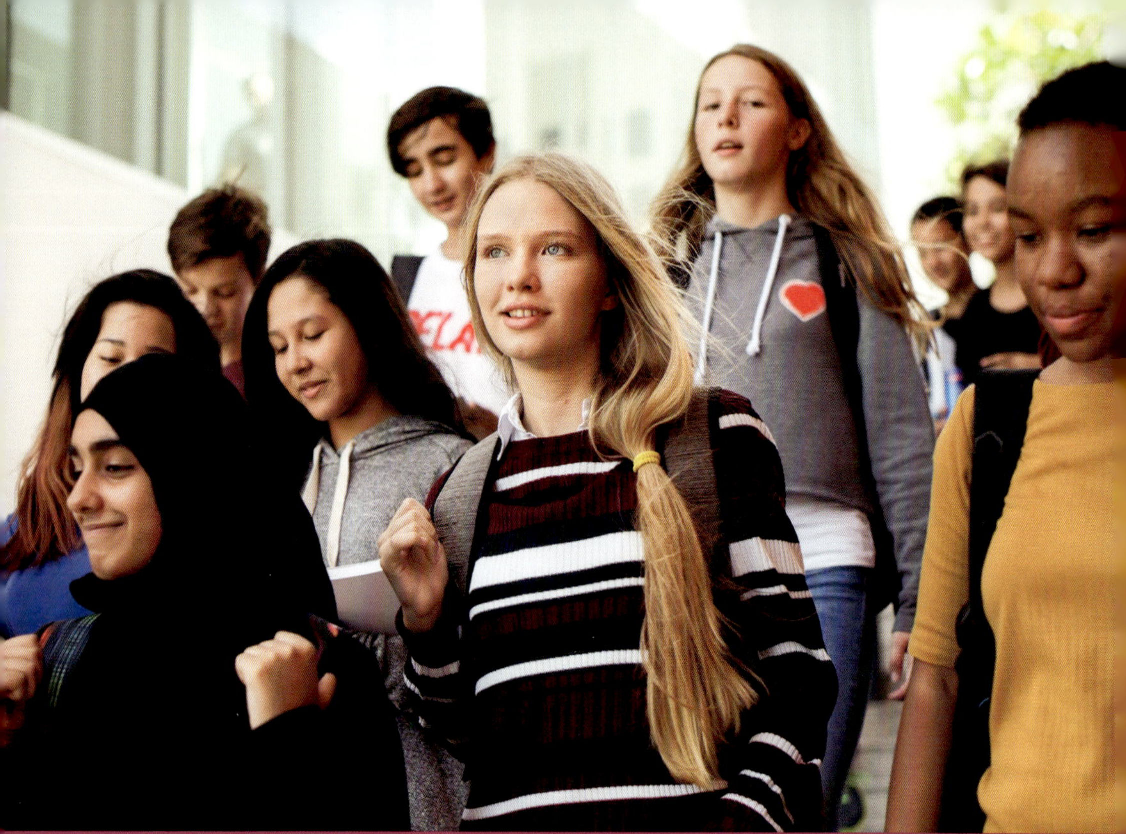

The neurodiversity movement encourages students and people around the world to celebrate different ways of thinking.

ASD to explore their intense interests in certain subjects.

Companies could eliminate job interviews for people with ASD. These people often do poorly in interviews because they do not make eye contact. People with ADHD do not do well in open offices. In those loud offices, they cannot focus on their work.

The neurodiversity movement wants to change the way people think about developmental disorders. These disorders can cause problems. But they also allow for special ways of thinking.

Today, many people with ASD, ADHD, and other developmental disorders no longer want to feel ashamed. They are proud of their differences. They want to celebrate what they can do for the world.

GLOSSARY

chronic

lasting for a long time or occurring over and over again

diagnosed

to have identified a medical condition by examining symptoms

genes

information in people's cells that determines traits such as height and eye color

hyperactivity

overactive and disruptive behavior

institutions

medical facilities that provide round-the-clock care for patients with mental or physical conditions

sterilized

to have medically prevented a person from being able to have children

stimulant

a medication or substance that increases activity in the brain and nervous system

toxins

substances that harm the body

SOURCE NOTES

INTRODUCTION: BEING DIFFERENT IS A SUPERPOWER

1. Quoted in Alison Rourke, "Greta Thunberg Responds to Asperger's Critics,'" *Guardian*, September 2, 2019. www.theguardian.com.

CHAPTER ONE: THE HISTORY OF DEVELOPMENTAL DISORDERS

2. Quoted in Klaus W. Lange et al., "The History of Attention Deficit Hyperactivity Disorder," *NCBI*, November 30, 2010. www.ncbi.nlm.nih.gov.

CHAPTER TWO: NOTABLE DEVELOPMENTAL DISORDERS

3. Quoted in Sandhya Somashekhar, "How Autistic Adults Banded Together to Start a Movement," *Washington Post*, July 20, 2015. www.washingtonpost.com.

4. Quoted in Kathryn Whitbourne, "What's It Really Like to Have ADHD?" *WebMD*, 2015. www.webmd.com.

CHAPTER THREE: DEVELOPMENTAL DISORDERS AND EVERYDAY LIFE

5. Quoted in Anahad O'Connor, "School Bullies Prey on Children with Autism," *New York Times*, September 3, 2012. https://well.blogs.nytimes.com.

CHAPTER FOUR: TREATING DEVELOPMENTAL DISORDERS

6. Quoted in Aimee Crawford, "Bravo, Simone Biles, for Taking a Stand Against ADHD Stigma," *ESPN*, September 21, 2016. www.espn.com.

7. Quoted in Somashekhar, "How Autistic Adults Banded Together to Start a Movement."

FOR FURTHER RESEARCH

BOOKS

Sue Bradford Edwards, *What Are Learning Disorders?* San Diego, CA: BrightPoint, 2023.

Carol Hand, *Handling ADHD.* Minneapolis, MN: Abdo, 2021.

Lindsey Sterling, *The Social Survival Guide for Teens on the Autism Spectrum.* Emeryville, CA: Rockridge, 2020.

INTERNET SOURCES

Mark Barna, "Everything Worth Knowing About . . . Autism Spectrum Disorder," *Discover,* June 19, 2017. www.discovermagazine.com.

Peter Jaksa, "I Can Do It Myself," *ADDitude,* September 21, 2021. www.additudemag.com.

Nicholette Zeliadt, "What Causes Autism?" *New York Times,* April 20, 2020. www.nytimes.com.

WEBSITES

American Association on Intellectual and Developmental Disabilities (AAIDD)
www.aaidd.org

AAIDD promotes research into ID and policies that protect the rights of people with intellectual disabilities.

Asperger/Autism Network (AANE)
www.aane.org

AANE provides information, practical advice, and support for people with autism and their families.

Children and Adults with Attention-Deficit/ Hyperactivity Disorder (CHADD)
https://chadd.org

CHADD offers information and resources for adults with ADHD, parents of children with ADHD, and specialists treating patients with the disorder.

INDEX

IMAGE CREDITS

Cover: © Pixel Head Photo/ iStockphoto
5: © The Visuals You Need/ Shutterstock Images
7: © Mike Dotta/Shutterstock Images
9: © Prostock Studio/ Shutterstock Images
10: © Juan Monino/iStockphoto
12: © Andras Csontos/ Shutterstock Images
15: © Andreas Mellentin/ Shutterstock Images
17: © Fat Camera/iStockphoto
19: © Satjawat Boontanataweepol/ iStockphoto
21: © Lopolo/Shutterstock Images
24: © DME Photography/iStockphoto
29: © Drazen/iStockphoto
31: © Tommaso 79/iStockphoto
32: © Elena Gromova Ru/ Shutterstock Images
37: © Janulla/iStockphoto
39: © Red Line Editorial
41: © FG Trade/iStockphoto
45: © Motortion Films/ Shutterstock Images
46: © Dr. Ake Krisda/ Shutterstock Images
49: © Wally Bird/Shutterstock Images
52: © Insta Photos/iStockphoto
55: © Victoria Gnatiuk/iStockphoto
56: © Monkey Business Images/ Shutterstock Images
59: © Monkey Business Images/ iStockphoto
60: © Nina Lishchuk/ Shutterstock Images
63: © Azman L./iStockphoto
66: © Prostock Studio/iStockphoto
68: © A. Ricardo/Shutterstock Images
72: © Raw Pixel/Shutterstock Images

ABOUT THE AUTHOR

Liz Sonneborn is a writer and editor. She is the author of more than one hundred nonfiction books for children, middle readers, and young adults. She specializes in biographies, US history, world history, Native American studies, and women's studies. A graduate of Swarthmore College, Sonneborn lives in Brooklyn, New York.